ME,
YOU,
AND
MEMORIES

ME, YOU, AND MEMORIES

A WAY TO HOLD

ALZHEIMER'S

AND DEMENTIA BACK

Denise M. Coravelli

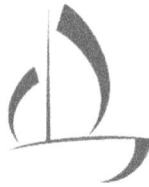

Ballast Books, LLC
www.ballastbooks.com

ISBN: 978-1-964934-59-4

Printed in Hong Kong

Cover Design by The Republic Factory
Layout by Suzanne Uchytil

Published by Ballast Books
www.ballastbooks.com

For more information, bulk orders, appearances, or speaking
requests, please email: info@ballastbooks.com

*Thank you to my family and friends, including my CMA
family and my football family,
for all your support.*

*To all individuals, family members, friends,
and caregivers affected by
Alzheimer's/dementia.*

I truly hope this helps you with your loved ones.

CONTENTS

AUTHOR'S NOTE

FIRST, LET ME START off by saying that I am not a doctor, and this is not a cure for Alzheimer's or dementia. It is a way to hold it back a year, two years, or maybe even three—hopefully more. Put simply, this book is meant to be a guide for the individual with Alzheimer's or dementia and their family. More than anything else, I hope this book offers a sense of hope and connection to those looking for support on their journey.

INTRODUCTION

In the year 2000, I boldly and decisively stepped out of the corporate world. To put it mildly, I decided it was time to take a little break. So I opened the newspaper to the classified ads, closed my eyes, and randomly poked at the open page in front of me. My finger—perhaps driven by fate—landed on a listing for the activities director in an assistant living facility.

What seemed like an arbitrary choice ended up drastically changing my life. As the activities director, I had the distinct pleasure of getting acquainted with seventy-five residents on an individual basis. Getting to know all the residents personally was amazing! Oh, the stories and history you can learn are unlike anything taught in school.

In my role, I created a daily, weekly, and monthly calendar for residents. I would meticulously plan out a week's worth of activities and read them out every day so the residents would know what to look forward to. Of course, these calendars were jam-packed with activities, including morning news, exercise sessions, movie nights, rummage sales, swap meets, socials with food, music events, Bible study and prayer groups, and so on. There were also clubs focusing on things like book sharing, chess, backgammon—you name it. And I can't forget the famous bingo night! We learned to do anything fun and safe to keep the residents stimulated. All of these activities were a great way to get family and caregivers involved too!

For example, one time, we put on a facility-wide fashion show. We put Christmas lights in the foyer area and made runways. Then, all the caregivers pitched in with each individual resident, going through their closet to pick out clothes for their debut on the runway. It was such a memorable occasion that brought such joy to the residents and the whole team!

Another activity that the residents loved was the pen pal program. We invited elementary school students to come in and form connections with the residents. Then, they would write to them throughout the year. The residents loved it. This program created an opportunity for them to share their wisdom with the younger generation and be a mentor to children who could look up to and love them.

I had so much fun with the residents in this position! I recall spotting a big van outside early on. It was a twelve-seater with a wheelchair lift. Right then and there, I knew that I wanted to learn how to drive it so I could assist with transportation to fun activities! I practiced until I could drive the residents around safely. From then on, we were able to take field trips, and the great kitchen team would make us lunches to go. So much fun! It was so wonderful to get the residents out of the facility and give them the chance to go on excursions.

It was my first time being an activities director, so it was a whole new world to me, and I learned so much—not just about the role but about life from the incredible humans I was engaging with.

Time passed swiftly, as it tends to do, and what was meant to be one year turned into four years.

Although I loved my job, not everything about it was perfect. Watching many of the residents get diagnosed with dementia or Alzheimer's was sad, especially when they had to leave the assisted facility to go to a specific memory care center. Unfortunately, once that happened, they would often decline much faster due to the major upheaval.

I witnessed this pattern many times, and it brought me a strangely pervasive sense of grief—but also ignited a firm resolve to make a positive difference for these extraordinary human beings whose minds were being stolen far too soon.

After my second year of seeing this and becoming very close with the residents, I asked the administrator if we could turn the first floor, which was the safest, into an Alzheimer's facility. We had three floors, and I thought this would be an excellent focus for that space.

They loved the idea! From there, I found myself being educated left and right. Determined to gather the knowledge and resources necessary to make this new goal happen, I attended every seminar that I could and ultimately learned so many incredible strategies to keep our residents in the facility that they were comfortable in.

In the end, my dream came to fruition. I was able to apply all that research and education to lead a phenomenal transformation. We created a beautiful and safe Alzheimer's/dementia facility on the first floor. It had an open environment where the residents could walk around. They had their own dining space as well as a communal area where they could sit and chat, knit, and do puzzles. Residents would even dance together! We also had a safe outdoor patio for the Alzheimer's/dementia residents to enjoy.

Of course, along with the physical changes to the floor, there were some changes to the way caregivers carried out their jobs. In fact, they had to receive special training to effectively communicate and work with residents. For example, if Jimmy wanted to send a package to his mom, we would simply say okay. We wouldn't remind them that their mom had passed away. We would just take the package somewhere else. In many ways, our goal was to facilitate friendships and promote longevity.

I am proud to say this is still going strong today! Residents were grateful for this opportunity, and they are still benefiting from this Alzheimer's/dementia facility. I am honored to have helped bring it to life.

During my time as the activities director, I very much considered the residents my family. When I got married, many residents attended the wedding, and when my first grandchild was born in 2002, they got to witness that and be part of the baby shower.

After those four years as activities director, three years after I launched the Alzheimer's/dementia facility on the first floor, I moved to Bozeman, Montana. I was proud of what I had accomplished, and at the same time, I was ready for a fresh start. During the eighteen years I lived in Montana, I worked with horses and decided to dabble in photography. I opened a modeling mentoring agency, CMA Modeling Agency, in 2010. I also mentored college football players in landscaping and restoration.

While in Montana, I was able to consult with many individuals diagnosed with Alzheimer's/dementia. This is when the word "Alzheimer's" became "Bruce"; the name was easier for them to remember. I was able to introduce the idea of holding "Bruce" back and facing him head-on by using brain exercises, along with physical exercise, to create better muscle stimulation and retention. I was able to develop a set of strategies for helping those living with Alzheimer's or dementia retain their sense of self for as long as possible.

Having the opportunity to try out my caregiving ideas led to the creation of this book, per a couple of individuals' requests. They encouraged me to share all of this since it had made such a difference in their lives.

With this book as a resource, I truly hope that you can find some way of holding Alzheimer's/dementia back with your beloved friends or someone close to you.

With all my heart,

Denise

Let's hold Bruce back!

(Sorry to anybody out there named Bruce. This is not meant to be a personal attack on your name. It's just a way of personifying Alzheimer's/dementia in a way that's easier to remember!)

EARLY
STAGE

MOST PEOPLE IN THE early stage of Alzheimer's or dementia still function relatively independently. In fact, they may still drive and even hold a job. Certainly, they may have a thriving social life. As a result, it may not be immediately obvious that Alzheimer's/dementia is taking hold. It's important to notice the little red flags here and there. The sooner you get a diagnosis, the sooner you can start fighting back against "Bruce." Then, you can turn to the Alzheimer's Association for helpful resources and educational tools to learn more about the disease and how to manage it.

Just like with any disease or disorder, attitude is crucial when it comes to prognosis. So most everyone who is diagnosed with Alzheimer's/dementia from the beginning would need to have the desire to take it on in order for the following strategies to make a true difference.

In addition, all parties need to be on the same page for positive results to follow—individuals with Alzheimer's/ dementia, their loved ones, and their other caretakers.

Here is a strategy that has worked wonders for the individuals I worked with, and I hope it will make a major difference for you too. It takes just two hours every morning. After medication is taken and breakfast is done, start with a nice chat. The goal is to know where your individual is at—mentally, physically, and emotionally—about one hour before you start your exercises. This will help you gauge the individual's current state and decide what you will be doing together that day.

Ultimately, this is always done together. You are the coach, and the individual is the player. It's a team effort, as you work toward a shared goal!

Once you've got a game plan, devote the first hour to working on your mental exercises using any mental app that you can find that fits your particular needs. Our personal favorite is Lumosity. I have been working with this app for over ten years and felt it was the best way to go. You can put in the person's birth date, and the games adjust to their age. It's perfect. However, some other options include Mind Mate and Constant Therapy. You should choose whatever app works best for you and the individual's needs and goals.

Be sure to explain the games to the individual with Alzheimer's or dementia. From there, you can establish and introduce to your loved one how to keep track of each game and each score. This will allow you to know if Bruce is showing himself or if you are holding him back—together.

To help you set the pace, try applying these tips for implementing the memory exercises:

You'll need to download the memory app on a Notepad, iPad, or other smart device big enough to see properly and move fingers and hands in swiping motions.

Before working with the individual with Alzheimer's/dementia, the person coaching should familiarize themselves with the games on their own device. Always keep your practice separate from the individual's device. That way, stats remain at the appropriate level for each age range.

Prepare a weekly stat sheet. This helps you both see where the individual with Alzheimer's/dementia is improving at the game as well as identify where there needs to be improvement.

Limit this phase to only five games a day with three attempts at each game. Be sure to take three- to five-minute breaks in between each game.

Make a homework sheet with the three lowest games. This can be worked on only if the person with Alzheimer's/dementia wants to later in the day after eating lunch and taking a nap. Mental rest is just as important as physical rest for these individuals.

In addition to leveraging memory apps like Lumosity, Mind Mate, and Constant Therapy, it's a good idea to use flashcards to stimulate the mind and help the person with Alzheimer's/dementia retain their memory as much as possible.

You can use flashcards depicting animals, vehicles, colors, fruits and vegetables, appliances—whatever you'd like. Pull out ten different cards each week to work with. Hold the flashcard for the individual and give them the opportunity to say what it is. If they are unable to vocalize the graphic on the flashcard, put it aside to work on after you go through all the rest. Basically, all the ones that were missed should go into the homework pile.

Speaking of homework, give the individual three simple words to study and remember for the next morning. An example might be truck, fork, and shovel. Then, the next morning, you will ask the individual to recall those three words and go over the worksheet (example in the back of the book) together. At that point, you'll discuss any frustration and turn everything into a positive. Encouraging words are always appreciated.

Keep in mind, empathy and understanding are key. Never argue and please do not talk to the individual like a child. Try to put yourself in their place. It's incredibly difficult to be battling your own mind on a daily basis! Compassion is everything.

After you've focused on mental exercises, devote the second hour to physical exercise. This can look different for different people. Of course, you'll want to consult your doctor to ensure you're only engaging in activities that are safe and healthy for you (or the person with Alzheimer's/dementia). However, some examples include walking, gardening, and even going out for different types of excursions like fishing, bowling, or whatever the individual likes.

Some more rigorous but supremely beneficial exercises include stair stepping, rubber band stretches, use of light hand weights, dancing, chair yoga, and so on. These help with balance and feet shuffling.

Here are some more specific examples of physical exercises you and your loved one can try:

Spend fifteen minutes using strength bands while seated or standing next to a chair for support.

Use an elliptical for fifteen minutes in three- to five-minute increments. This will help with picking feet up if you notice shuffling when walking. It will also help prevent tripping and make it easier for the individual to go up or down steps. Of course, make sure you're nearby or spotting the person just in case.

Take a walk if the weather is nice. Just going for a stroll is great for you and the person living with Alzheimer's/dementia!

Dancing freestyle or taking structured dance lessons are always fun options. Music is a beautiful, healing, and happy mood tool. Plus, dancing is good for socializing.

In general, find fun activities to enjoy together. Get to know what the individual likes to do and go do those things. Happy endorphins are good for the brain!

It's all about determining an exercise regimen that will keep the individual as healthy and fit as possible from a physical standpoint. After all, physical and mental health go hand in hand! Once you develop a routine filled with exercises the person with Alzheimer's/dementia enjoys, you'll be able to establish a great relationship characterized by trust and fun. Of course, my wish for you is much laughter or many hugs when needed!

Spending two hours a day on mental and physical exercise can make a huge difference for your loved one, but there are plenty of other best practices you can keep in mind to improve their health throughout the day:

Prioritize mental and physical rest. Find a time after lunch to make sure your loved one takes a nap. One to two hours of sleep during the day is ideal. This allows the brain to rest and helps with improving clarity and speaking. Then, going to bed at an ideal time and getting at least six to seven hours of sleep make a huge difference.

Eating healthy foods to fuel the brain is important as well. Research foods that support neurological health. Brain stimulation foods would be helpful for anyone, including you! Make sure to have a nutritious breakfast, such as oatmeal. Blueberries and acai are phenomenal, so perhaps mix those in. It's all about transforming food from being a comfort thing to being something healthy and also fun.

A helpful suggestion is to allow the individual to choose their favorites from the healthy options. Remember, it's important to allow the individual to still exert independence and make choices for themselves so they don't think they have to rely on somebody else. They're still the boss!

Most individuals are on medication. Taking the meds thirty minutes prior to exercises and having breakfast is ideal.

Overall, following a routine is extremely important. If you don't follow a healthy daily routine, your loved one with Alzheimer's/dementia will definitely decline at a faster pace.

Always be a safe place for the person you are caring for.

If agitation starts to show, it's vital to learn how to redirect in a positive way. Sometimes just listening and saying you understand helps. For example, asking "How can I help you?" can calm the individual and make them feel comfortable and cared about too.

Here's something else to consider. If you're out and about, and suddenly, another person wants to tell the individual that they are wrong about something, the person correcting them has embarrassed the person with Alzheimer's. In all likelihood, they have made your loved one agitated. The person living with dementia may even start to act nasty.

In that case, you can redirect by saying, "Oh my goodness, can you help me with something? Can you help me understand what we were talking about yesterday? I can't remember what you told me about your mom. Where was she born?"

Why? It's all about empowerment and reminding the person with Alzheimer's/dementia of a positive memory.

Of course, it's helpful to know the individual to do that. If you don't know them, and you're just a bystander, and they go off for some reason—there's too much noise in the restaurant, the waitress said the wrong thing, they're struggling to get their words out properly—instead of trying to fill in the words for them, redirect them to something you know is simple.

"How is your steak? Do you need more water? Would you like to join me for a walk outside? I need a bit of fresh air."

You're the (re)director, but you want to word it in such a way that they feel they are calling the shots. The goal is to establish that independence and let them know they're helping you rather than the other way around. Ask a better question, keep it positive, and ask for help. That's the key to successfully redirecting.

I also want to emphasize how important a safety list is. I highly encourage you to create a room-to-room checklist for your loved one. It might include items like lights off, water off, stove off, and heaters monitored. Are things in the way? Can they hurt themselves? Everyone's checklist will be different, but it's important to have some routine process in place to ensure the safety of your loved one in their space.

The early stage is a difficult time for everyone—especially for our loved ones dealing with Bruce rearing his ugly head and being a bully. Not being able to control certain thoughts like they used to is understandably upsetting and can even be embarrassing. Remember, it's not their fault, and they need to lovingly be reminded of that.

Finally, be patient and don't be afraid to ask for help. Caregiver burnout is a real thing. Your mental and physical well-being are important too, so if you are struggling or have concerns about the person you're caring for, take action—for you and your loved one.

As you've undoubtedly noticed, the main theme of this chapter is exercise. As they say, "use it or lose it." That's why it's so important to incorporate these mental and physical exercises on a daily basis. They are key to holding Bruce back!

MIDDLE
STAGES

THE MIDDLE STAGES OF Alzheimer's/dementia can last the longest time—often many years. You may only notice small differences at first, but these changes will progress over time, and this will correlate to a greater level of care for the individual.

It may start with them having a hard time focusing. If you see this happening, then it's best to slow down. Turn off or move away from any distracting background sounds, such as TV, music, or other people talking.

From there, you may note poorer retention. For example, your loved one may forget the structure or routine of the games that you play every day. They may start to ask "Why?" a lot more often. Or they might say things like, "No, it's not like this—it should be like this," trying to convince themselves that they're not forgetting something.

They may even begin to stutter a bit, which can be frustrating to them.

My tip to you? Don't watch them be embarrassed. You might not want to go out as much to prevent them from experiencing a sense of mortification. They may even say they don't like the game anymore to avoid the situation. However, as the caregiver, your focus should be to try to stay as strong as possible. Offer to write out the instructions to help them stay as self-sufficient as possible for as long as possible. We'll talk more about this later!

Notice if the individual is tired. Maybe they didn't get enough rest the night before. If that's the case, then perhaps take an early break and have them go lie down for a little nap. After they've rested for at least one hour, resume your activities and exercises as normal.

All in all, everything from the early stages will pretty much stay the same except for you'll be learning more patience as the caregiver or coach. It's still going to be important to make sure that the individual with Alzheimer's/dementia takes their medication, eats a nutritious breakfast, and gets whatever rest they need before doing the exercises. Then, just as you did during the early stage, start by having a simple conversation to gauge the individual's headspace. Is Bruce showing his ugly self? Engaging with the person you're caring for should help you understand where they are mentally and emotionally.

Once you're ready to dive in and start the morning, it may take a little longer than it normally did during the early stage. However, it's still going to be productive, and your earnest efforts will make the individual feel like they have made a great accomplishment. What an awesome way to start the day! And you're playing a key role in that for the person with Alzheimer's/dementia.

Remember that endorphins are excellent for you and the individual you're caring for, so getting outside or putting on some music and dancing is always a good time. They may not be able to pursue the same activities they always loved as the Alzheimer's/dementia progresses, so maintain an open dialogue to determine how to best engage with them physically and mentally. Perhaps they can't go bowling or take long walks anymore, but they really enjoy cooking or gardening. Hobbies such as painting, card games, board games, large and simple word-find puzzles, puzzles with big pieces, watching movies, or simply just talking about fun things in the past by looking through photo books can make a positive difference. It's all about being adaptable based on the changing needs of the individual while still incorporating the things that bring them joy in new and creative ways.

During the middle stages, it's not uncommon for someone living with Alzheimer's/dementia to struggle with completing everyday tasks that they never had trouble with in the past. As their condition progresses, it can be difficult for them to remember how to perform certain actions or use certain things.

I have found that creating a simple how-to book is a great way for an individual to exert their independence without having to constantly ask for help. I call this a reminder book, a phrase that I put in big, bold letters on the front of the binder. I start off with pictures of things like a remote control on the left side. Then, on the right side, I provide an example of what buttons to use, how to use them, and what they do. I simply cross out the buttons that no longer need to be pushed on the remote control. Then, I do the same for telephones, the thermostat, the washer and dryer, the microwave, and so on.

Everyone's reminder book will be different. After all, every person's environment is unique, and your how-to book will be customized based on your loved one's home. Just capture all the items and tasks the individual with Alzheimer's/dementia uses on a regular basis, and soon, your book will be filled with a plethora of critical information that will help the person navigate independently for as long as possible.

Keep in mind, if the individual is on their laptop or cell phone a lot, eventually, their brain will start to get exhausted from constantly pushing buttons and seeing the advertisements or the distracting spam mail that comes in. This, unfortunately, will distract and confuse the individual and Bruce will definitely rear his ugly head.

A wonderful solution for this is to set a specific time slot for the person to be on their laptop or cell phone. It's also a good practice to also encourage the individual to look up from their smart device and glance around at their surroundings periodically during this allotted time frame so their eyes and brain don't get too tired. Then, when the time slot comes to an end, gently suggest that it's time to consider putting the technology down to take a little rest. They can always pick it up again later.

Now, be very mindful about how you make this suggestion. No one likes to be talked down to or told what to do, and someone living with Alzheimer's/dementia is no different. It's vital that you treat each individual with respect the way that you would want to be treated, so it's best to make it the individual's choice so they still feel like an adult.

One way to do this respectfully is to create two suggestions so they feel in control but still are prompted to pursue a course of action that's healthy for them. For example, you could say, "It's totally your choice—when would you like to take a nap? At one o'clock or at three o'clock?" Once they pick a time, you just remind them that you'll be back at one o'clock or three o'clock to help get them ready. From there, you can offer another set of options: "Would you prefer to rest here on the couch or in your bedroom?" It's all about empowering them to make decisions for themselves so they don't feel constrained by their Alzheimer's/dementia.

While navigating this conversation, in an effort to help them get the mental and physical rest they need, it also helps to remove the laptop out of the view of the individual. Don't just pick it up and move it without consulting them. Help them be a part of the decision by asking them if you can put the laptop or other smart device away so it's not a distraction during their resting time.

After lunch is a perfect time to lie down and watch a movie, read a book, or listen to some soothing music before the individual falls asleep. Even if they never actually nod off, having the opportunity to gently let their brain relax will set them up for success for the rest of the day.

Caregivers, it's very important that you find some relaxation time also! This is your chance to unwind as well so that you're ready to be hands on with helping your loved one again in the afternoon or the next day—whatever the case may be.

LATE
STAGE

The LATE STAGE OF Alzheimer's/dementia captures the period of time when the disease has progressed exponentially. Often, an individual at this stage may require intensive, around-the-clock care.

When an individual enters the late stage, you'll notice what will look and sound like stuttering, or the mouth and lips will quiver when the person is trying to get their words out. This leads to a common misconception. Often, when this happens, people will say, "Oh my gosh, they are getting much worse." Yes, the disease is progressing, but just because the individual can't say the word does not mean they don't know it. Bruce is rearing his ugly head again and not allowing the words to come out. Their brain still knows it—the word is just locked inside. Your loved one is still there and still the person you care about.

Try to view the situation from your loved one's perspective. If they're really struggling to get words out, their frustration is sure to increase. You may feel frustrated too, but don't push them. Learn to be selfless and make sacrifices for your loved ones. It shouldn't even be a sacrifice! It's done out of love. For instance, if you usually go to restaurants, but it's starting to be overwhelming to your loved one, cut it down. Don't go out as often. Routine is more crucial than ever at this point, so ensure your loved one gets the structure they need.

For example, one time, one of the individuals I was working with started having challenges with verbally identifying the pictures on his flashcards. I could see the frustration and a bit of defeat in his demeanor. It was then that I had the idea of enhancing the flashcards and using them as a tool to help him communicate when his brain wouldn't let him find the word he was looking for.

To do this, I put the words describing the flashcards on large laminated white strips. Once that was done, I put all the laminated words out on the table and then held up one flashcard at a time. As soon as I showed a card, he would grab the right word—and he was 100 percent correct. I knew he could do it!

The look on his face and the satisfaction that he derived from being able to complete this seemingly simple but hugely significant task was paramount. The fact that he could make this identification without frustration allowed him to feel proud again, and his sense of accomplishment and empowerment went beyond what he or anyone else could describe in words. He was so happy with himself, and that, in turn, brought me immense joy. I will admit there were some tears in my eyes, and I experienced great satisfaction for him and for me.

You see, every individual with Alzheimer's/dementia who is trying to express themselves may not be able to say the words, but they know what they want to say. It is crucial to be patient with each individual and with yourself. There's always a way to find out how to communicate better for those who can't express themselves the way they'd like to.

Keeping things simple helps those living with Alzheimer's/dementia, and the caregivers and the family members too.

There will come a time when traveling or even going out to dinner or the movies will become very agitating to those with Alzheimer's/dementia. Something that seemed to be pretty straightforward and that gave the person pleasure may not anymore. That's okay—it's part of this disease. You shouldn't try to force your loved one to continue doing those things, and you shouldn't allow any frustration or disappointment you feel to drive the way you interact with them.

Here's an anecdote to put this into perspective for you. Eight months ago, I watched somebody travel with her husband who had dementia. To my dismay, I noticed they were arguing and getting frustrated in the airport. It was so hurtful to witness, especially since I knew what this gentleman must have been going through—and what his wife was going through. There's no doubt that navigating Alzheimer's/dementia is incredibly difficult for both the person living with it and the caregivers and loved ones.

The lesson here is, at some point, you just have to stop arguing and snapping for the sake of peace and harmony. It's better for both you and the individual with Alzheimer's/dementia.

No matter how dedicated you are to caring for your loved one, there's a strong likelihood that you will have to move them to a memory care center or hire a twenty-four-hour homecare service at some point during this process, whether it's in the early or late stages. Regardless of the timing, make sure you really do your homework when selecting a facility or at-home caretaker. It's crucial that you feel confident that the ones caring for your family member will truly protect them and have their best interests at heart.

Be aware of those who prey on the elderly. If you suspect this of anyone, whether it be a stranger, a friend, or even a family member, take appropriate action. There are resources for just such circumstances. If you feel someone is taking advantage of your loved one or they are being neglected or suffering any form of elder abuse—including financial abuse—this should be reported to your local Adult Protective Services (APS) office immediately.

All in all, I feel it's very important to also remain close by for the safety of the individual with Alzheimer's/dementia. This is most important during sundowning, which, as the name suggests, happens most often at night. The signs may include increased confusion or anxiety and behaviors such as pacing, wandering, or yelling.

Remember, as you navigate the late stage of Alzheimer's/dementia, it's crucial to cherish each and every day and moment with your loved one. You can make it a great day, even if it's a bad day. Keep in mind, these days together unfortunately won't last much longer. It's important to truly treasure every bit of time you get together before it's gone.

As the days become weeks, the weeks become months, and the months become years, there will come a point when memories start to diminish, especially the short-term ones. The individual with Alzheimer's/dementia will most likely go into a memory—a year when they were the happiest.

Don't try to bring them back to your present. Let them live in their "present." Allow them to linger there where they are happy for the moment. Ask questions like, "What year is it? I forgot. Can you help me remember?" When the individual tells you what year it is, that will help you understand where they are in their mind. Remember, don't correct them. Let them be happy. Let them share that happiness with you. As long as the individual with Alzheimer's/dementia is willing to continue to exercise and follow a wonderful routine, then enjoy the moments with them as long as you can.

Once the person has lost the memory of who exactly you are or the things that you used to do with them, it will likely be devastating to you. But remember, it's often harder on the family members, friends, or caregivers than it is on the individual with Alzheimer's/dementia. Yes, there is no cure for Alzheimer's right now, but God gave them a gift. They don't remember, so they don't have to be so frustrated and embarrassed. They are free to enjoy the best moments from their life. Even though Bruce has, in many ways, taken over, your loved one is able to move freely through their memories and live in whatever moments brought them the most joy and fulfillment.

This is an opportunity for you too. When your loved one reverts back to a different period of their lives in their mind, you have the chance to learn things you never knew before about them. You can catch a glimpse into their beautiful, amazing life.

The main thing to remember is that your loved one doesn't have to battle anymore once they reach the final stage—they can just live. And as hard as that may be for you, as the caregiver, for them, it is truly a blessing.

Let them live in their new world of peace. I hope that you will find some peace in that too.

RESOURCES

THE NEXT PAGES PROVIDE pictures and descriptions of key resources, including samples of the brain exercise sheet that you'll use with the app you choose to download.

Flashcards & Namecards

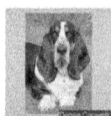

Dog

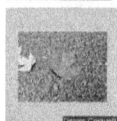

Leaf

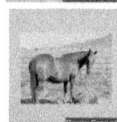

Horse

Denise Coravelli

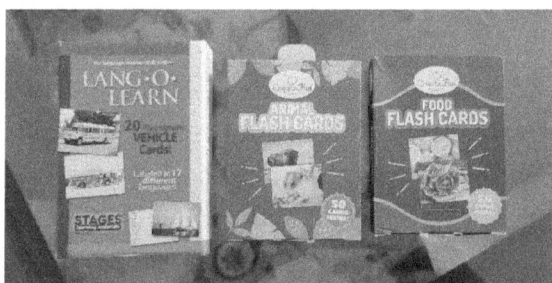

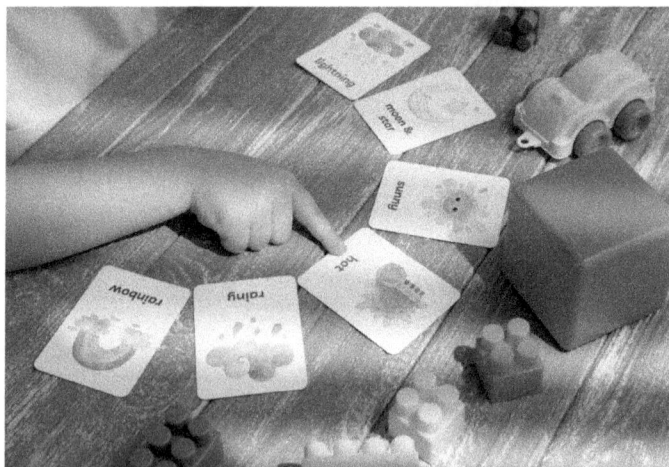

MONTREAL COGNITIVE ASSESSMENT (MOCA)
Version 7.1 Original Version

NAME :
Education :   Date of birth :
Sex :   DATE :

VISUOSPATIAL / EXECUTIVE

Copy cube

Draw CLOCK (Ten past eleven)
(3 points)

POINTS

[ ]   [ ]   [ ] [ ] [ ]   /5
                     Contour Numbers Hands

NAMING

[ ]   [ ]   [ ]   /3

MEMORY

Read list of words, subject must repeat them. Do 2 trials, even if 1st trial is successful. Do a recall after 5 minutes.

	FACE	VELVET	CHURCH	DAISY	RED
1st trial					
2nd trial					

No points

ATTENTION

Read list of digits (1 digit/ sec.). Subject has to repeat them in the forward order   [ ] 2 1 8 5 4
Subject has to repeat them in the backward order   [ ] 7 4 2   /2

Read list of letters. The subject must tap with his hand at each letter A. No points if ≥ 2 errors
[ ] F B A C M N A A J K L B A F A K D E A A A J A M O F A A B   /1

Serial 7 subtraction starting at 100   [ ] 93   [ ] 86   [ ] 79   [ ] 72   [ ] 65
4 or 5 correct subtractions: 3 pts, 2 or 3 correct: 2 pts, 1 correct: 1 pt, 0 correct: 0 pt   /3

LANGUAGE

Repeat : I only know that John is the one to help today. [ ]
The cat always hid under the couch when dogs were in the room. [ ]   /2

Fluency / Name maximum number of words in one minute that begin with the letter F   [ ] _____ (N ≥ 11 words)   /1

ABSTRACTION

Similarity between e.g. banana - orange = fruit   [ ] train - bicycle   [ ] watch - ruler   /2

DELAYED RECALL

Has to recall words WITH NO CUE	FACE [ ]	VELVET [ ]	CHURCH [ ]	DAISY [ ]	RED [ ]	Points for UNCUED recall only	/5
Optional	Category cue						
	Multiple choice cue						

ORIENTATION

[ ] Date   [ ] Month   [ ] Year   [ ] Day   [ ] Place   [ ] City   /6

© Z.Nasreddine MD   www.mocatest.org   Normal ≥ 26 / 30   TOTAL   /30
Administered by _____   Add 1 point if ≤ 12 yr edu

Grit TO Grid

Grit to Grid was created by Krystle Saatjian, a certified dementia practitioner in Bozeman, Montana. A personal friend of Denise, Krystle is a natural at this work—compassionate, calming, and beautiful inside and out. Grit to Grid offers personalized word searches in large text that are laminated so they can be used again and again. Anyone can order these workbooks by visiting the Grit to Grid website.

https://www.grittogrid.org/

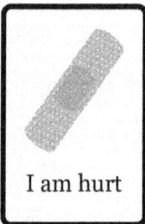

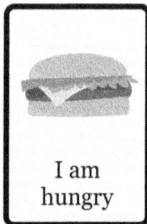

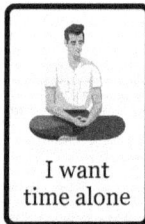

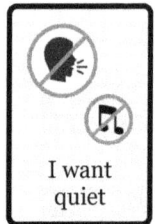

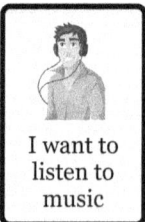

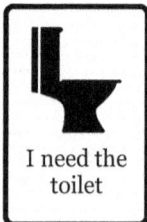

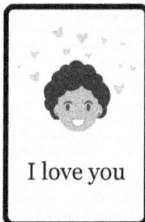

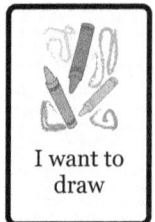

I am hurt	I am hungry	I want time alone	I want quiet
I want to listen to music	I need the toilet	I love you	I want to draw

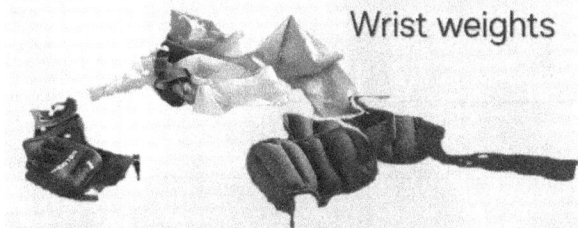

Chair exercises
Stretch bands
Ankle weights
Wrist weights

Denise Coravelli

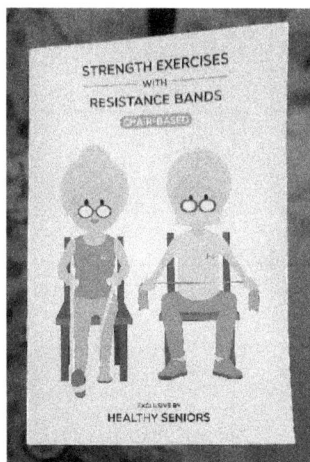

STRENGTH EXERCISES
— WITH —
RESISTANCE BANDS
CHAIR-BASED

HEALTHY SENIORS

Luminosity Worksheet (created by Denise)

Date	Catagory	Game	Score	Score	Score	Comments

At least two games per day.
No more than 5.

PARTING
THOUGHTS

THANK YOU FOR JOINING me on this journey by reading *Me, You, and Memories*. I was privileged to be able to work with individuals with Alzheimer's/dementia for so long. It is something that I always wanted to do, and I'm so happy that they gave me the opportunity to do these exercises with them. Now, I am passing those exercises on to you with the hope that this brings peace and positivity to you and your family when it comes to holding "Bruce" back.

—*Denise Coravelli*